Roberto Carlos Negreiros de Arruda et al.

OCCURRENCE OF ENDOPARASITES IN CAPYBARAS IN MARANHÃO

Roberto Carlos Negreiros de Arruda et al.

OCCURRENCE OF ENDOPARASITES IN CAPYBARAS IN MARANHÃO

Guidelines for educational purposes and the preservation or control of the species

ScienciaScripts

Imprint
Any brand names and product names mentioned in this book are subject to trademark, brand or patent protection and are trademarks or registered trademarks of their respective holders. The use of brand names, product names, common names, trade names, product descriptions etc. even without a particular marking in this work is in no way to be construed to mean that such names may be regarded as unrestricted in respect of trademark and brand protection legislation and could thus be used by anyone.

Cover image: www.ingimage.com

This book is a translation from the original published under ISBN 978-3-639-89883-5.

Publisher:
Sciencia Scripts
is a trademark of
Dodo Books Indian Ocean Ltd. and OmniScriptum S.R.L publishing group

120 High Road, East Finchley, London, N2 9ED, United Kingdom
Str. Armeneasca 28/1, office 1, Chisinau MD-2012, Republic of Moldova, Europe
Managing Directors: Ieva Konstantinova, Victoria Ursu
info@omniscriptum.com

Printed at: see last page
ISBN: 978-620-8-39501-8

SUMMARY

CHAPTER I

OCCURRENCE OF ENDOPARASITES IN FREE-LIVING CAPYARAS (HYDROCHOERUS HYDROCHAERIS) IN MARANHÃO

Roberto Carlos Negreiros de Arruda, Daniel Praseres Chaves, Viviane Correa Silva Coimbra, Francisco Borges Costa, Hermes Ribeiro Luz, José Hyrton Dantas Carneiro Júnior, Nádia Oliveira Medeiros, Karlos Yuri Fernandes Pedrosa, Valter Marchão Costa Filho, Robert Ferreira Barroso de Carvalho, Rafael Michael Silva Nogueira, Mylena Andréa oliveira Torres and Hamilton Pereira Santos

SUMMARY

The capybara is the largest rodent in the world, found in South and Central America, and one of its peculiarities is that its name derives from the Tupi-Guarani "kapibara", which means "grass eater", so Hydrochoerus hydrochaeris is a herbivore that eventually uses coprophagy and/or caecotrophy, However, there are still few reports in the literature about its intestinal microbiota, although zoonotic parasites such as Plagorchis muris, Neobalantidium coli, Cryptosporidium spp and Giardia spp have been identified circulating in capybaras. The aim of this study was to determine the occurrence of the main endoparasites of free-living capybaras in Maranhão. Thus, between February and October 2021, 37 fresh faecal samples were collected in four municipalities in the state of Maranhão: Balsas, Caxias, Itapecuru Mirim and Lima Campos for parasitological analyses. The Willis-Mollay (1921) and Faust (1939) methods were used to provide sedimentation of residues and spontaneous flotation of eggs and oocysts. The results showed that there was polyparasitism in the capybaras, since there were parasites present in the samples from all the municipalities, i.e. at least one specimen per positive sample. Thus, eggs of nematodes from the superfamilies Trichostrongyloidea (67.57%) and Trichuroidea (eggs of Capillaria sp in 5.41%), the Strongyloididae family (eggs of Strongyloides sp in 8.11%) and protozoa, oocysts of the genus Eimeria (32.43%) were detected. It was concluded that parasitism by nematodes and protozoa reveals the capybara's potential for endoparasitic maintenance, and possibly as a disseminator of these agents to domestic animals, wild animals and humans, whether in peri-urban or rural areas, in environments with an abundance of contaminated water, This brings us to a deeper analysis of the importance of veterinarians and other agricultural professionals in the theme of 'One Health', taking into account the biological cycles of parasites, ecology, pathology in species and their zoonotic potential.

INTRODUCTION

Capybaras belong to the Class Mammalia, Order Rodentia and Family Caviidae, specifically in the group of the largest rodents, as well as being rustic and neotropical herbivores, present in South and Central America, or rather, from northern Argentina to Panama, with a preference for low-lying or flooded areas (FORERO- MONTAÑA et al... 2003; MOREIRA et al, 2013), 2003; MOREIRA et al, 2013), in Tupi-Guarani "kapibara" means "grass eater" and they are also gregarious, as they live in groups with a dominant male, several females, young individuals and subordinate males (COSTA et al., 2002).

They live for ten to twelve years on the banks of rivers and lakes in family clusters, and use the water as protection and a hiding place from attack, especially from carnivores, and it is in this aquatic environment that all their vital activities take place, such as temperature control, hydration and reproduction (MACDONALD, 1981; ALVES, 2010). The capybara has a high fertility and fecundity rate (GONZÁLEZ- JIMÉNEZ, 1995). The female's gestation period is 150 days, with litters ranging from 1 to 8 cubs, or an average of 4 cubs per birth, with the possibility of 2 (two) births per year, and they also provide a high survival rate for the weaned young (HOSKEN & SILVEIRA; COSTA et al., 2002).

In areas with a high density of capybaras, they can compete with livestock for forage, invade and destroy crops, as well as deteriorating the quality of the water supply for domestic animals (FORERO-MONTAÑA et al., 2003), and on average they disperse between 3.4 and 5.6 kilometres, mainly due to feeding (HERRERA, 1992; HERRERA et al., 2013).

Capybaras carry a wide range of haemoparasites and intestinal parasites (MONES & MARTINEZ, 1982), and there is little specific literature on protozoa or helminths (nematodes, cestodes and trematodes) in their digestive tract or organs (CUETO, 2013). The Amazon rainforest, the Cerrado and the flooded savannas are examples of biomes that suffer from constant fires and the removal of native forests. The Maranhão Amazon, for example, has an average of 570 trees per hectare, where 109 species of fish, 124 mammals and 503 birds have been catalogued, all at risk due to the high levels of deforestation (MOURÃO, 2022). As a result of deforestation in the state, the number of H. hydrochaeris has been increasing as a result of the disappearance of their predators, mainly jaguars, caimans, anacondas and others. due to the prolificacy of the species. In this sense, it is possible that they are reservoirs and disseminators of parasites among domestic herds, and zoonotic diseases in this local interrelationship. The aim of this survey was to determine the occurrence of the main endoparasites of free-living H. hydrochaeris in Maranhão and their impact on 'unique health'.

MATERIAL AND METHODS

Stool parasitological tests

A total of 37 faecal samples were collected from free-living capybaras in the state of Maranhão between February and October 2021. The samples were collected near bodies of water (rivers, lakes and fish farm ponds) and packed in plastic bags or 50 mL conical collectors (tubes), in the proportion of seven to ten pellets from a mound of faeces, stored under refrigeration at 4-8°C. Most of the samples were fresh (bright olive colour) and were collected in areas where domestic animals, wild animals and peri-urban areas live together, with the most notable being the surrounding dry areas, in the following municipalities and sites: in the municipality of Caxias (peri-urban area), in Lima Campos (peri-urban area), in Itapecuru Mirim (rural area) and in Balsas/MA (rural area), the latter, further south in the state, which is very important for grain production, mainly soya and maize. Of the 04 (four) samples from the Lima Campos reservoir, 03 (three) faeces were drier or older, and of the 21 from Balsas, in 01 (one) sample, the syllables had a pasty appearance, which is believed to be diarrhoea in individual no. 09. The other faeces were considered new or moist. The study area points to four municipalities geolocalised on Google Earth, where capybaras had been monitored, to delimit the clusters of animals sampled as can be seen in subsequent georeferenced spatial maps (figures 1 and 2). Parasitological analyses took place at the CERNITAS Laboratory in São Luís - MA, using the Willis-Mollay (1921) and Faust (1939) methods, by sedimentation of residues and spontaneous flotation of eggs and oocysts, and the results were compiled in an Excel table and presented in frequencies by percentage. The captures and monitoring of capybaras in the field were authorised by the Ministry of the Environment - MMA, through the Chico Mendes Institute for Biodiversity Conservation - ICMBio, issued by the

Authorisation and Information System in Biodiversity - SISBIO, under no. 83484, as well as approved by the Ethics in Animal Experimentation Committee (EEA) of the State University of Maranhão (UEMA), under no. 030/2021-01200.002200/2015-06 CEEA/CMV/UEMA.

RESULTS AND DISCUSSION

There was polyparasitism in the capybaras of Maranhão, i.e. at least one species of parasite per positive sample, so a frequency of 100% (37/37) was obtained, where 81% (30/37) were parasitised by helminths and 32% (12/37) by protozoa of the genus Eimeria. Results with lower frequencies occurred in the analyses of 113 faecal samples in seven cities in São Paulo, where 97% (110/113) tested positive for the presence of helminth eggs and/or protozoan oocysts. They added that capybaras from anthropised areas had a higher species richness of endoparasites (SOUZA et al., 2021).

Figures 1 and 2 show the four municipalities georeferenced on the Google Earth map, where the capybaras were being visually monitored in order to delimit the clusters of animals sampled.

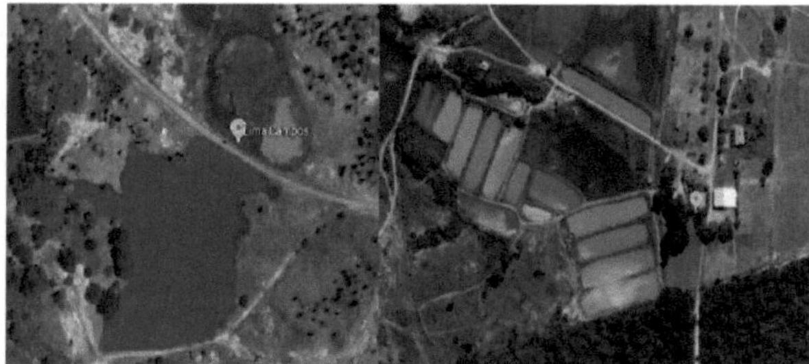

Figure 1: Collection locations shown in yellow pins on Google Earth (2021), the first near a lagoon in Lima Campos/MA, and the second near fishponds in Balsas/MA.

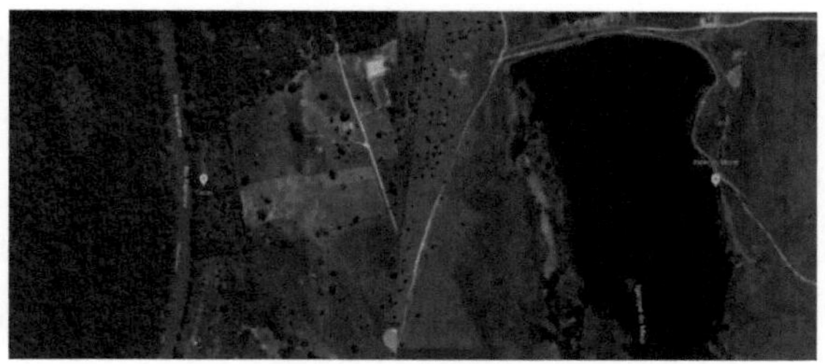

Figure 2: Locations of the collections shown in yellow pins on Google Earth, the third near the Itapecuru River in Caxias/MA, image on the left, and the fourth, in Itapecuru Mirim on the banks of a lagoon on the right.

In a total of 37 samples, 81% (30/37) had nematode eggs. Among these samples, 68% (25/37) had eggs from the Trichostrongyloidea superfamily, 5% (2/37) for the Trichuroidea (Capillaria sp.), and 8% (3/37) from the Strongyloididae family (Strongyloides sp.). The presence of protozoan oocysts (Eimeria sp.) in the samples was 32% (12/37). The data is shown in Table 1 and Figures 3 and 4.

Table 1. Frequency of endoparasites of free-living capybaras in different locations in Maranhão and percentage from February to October 2021.

Municipalities	No. of Samples		Helminths		Protozoa
		Superfamily		Family	Gender
		Trichostrongyloidea	Trichuroidea	Stongyloididae	Eimeria
Balsas	21	15 (71,43%)	2 (9,52%)	1 (4,76%)	9 (24,32%)
Caxias	4	3 (75,00%)	0 (0,00%)	1 (25,00%)	0 (0,00%)
Itapecuru Young	8	5 (62,50%)	0 (0,00%)	0 (0,00%)	2 (25,00%)
Lima Fields	4	2 (50,00%)	0 (0,00%)	1 (25,00%)	1 (25,00%)
Total	37	25 (67,77%)	2 (5,41%)	3 (8,11%)	12 (32,43%)

Similar results with the Trichostrongyloidea superfamily were highlighted by Sinkoc et al. (2009) and Souza et al. (2021), noting that the occurrence of nematodes Trichostrongylus axei, Haemonchus sp. and Cooperia spp. is considered accidental (SINKOC et al., 2009) and infection by these endoparasites in capybaras generally occurs in anthropised areas and requires cohabitation with livestock species that are managed and interact with humans, such as cattle, goats, sheep and horses (SOUZA et al., 2021). In a literature review, Alves et al. (2010) described coprophagia, which is the consumption of faeces on the ground, and cecotrophagia, which is the consumption of faeces from the rectum, as a way of making better use of food (high protein and vitamin value). Mendes et al. (2000) mention that this practice is widely observed in lagomorphs and other rodents. It is believed that this eventual habit is easier to observe in captivity.

Further studies should be carried out to see if coprophagy in some individuals or groups would explain the high rate of parasitism (polyparasitism) found in the Maranhão findings, and if there is a certain degree of resistance of some animal categories to these endoparasites, considering the adult animals of the species, for example, Costa & Catto (1994) observed a higher prevalence of Strongyloides chapini in young animals (91%) than in adults (9%).

Another perspective is the high temperatures near the aquatic environment, which favour parasites and infections, and it is also understood that capybaras serve as parasitological reservoirs for other species, by cohabiting or living together, especially with herbivores, as well as becoming a greater danger during the dry period of the year, due to the scarcity of pastures and greater contact between species.

An example of this coexistence is the Pantanal region of southern Mato Grosso, where cattle, deer, wild pigs, capybaras and other wild animals share the same environments (FONTANA, 2011). These production species were also seen in the Maranhão study area.

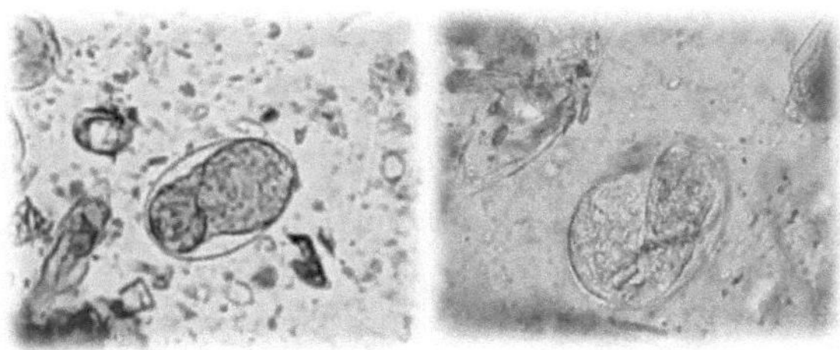

Figure 3. On the left is an egg of the Trichostrongyloidea superfamily and on the right is an egg of Strongyloides sp. (Strongyloididae family). Photos: Chaves, 2021.

In Juiz de Fora/MG, Vieira et al. (2006), classifying eggs and larvae of Strongyloides sp, identified it as Strongyloides chapini, since since the work of Sandground (1925), it had always been the only species of Rhabditida nematode that occurred in capybaras. Therefore, the findings from Maranhão may be Strongyloides chapini, although further studies are needed to confirm this.

Bonuti et al. (2002), studying 14 helminths in capybaras in the Pantanal of Mato Grosso do Sul, found Trichostrongylus axei (Trichostrongylidae) and Capillaria hydrochoeri (Trichuridae). Sinkoc et al. (2004), evaluating the occurrence of parasitic helminths in the gastrointestinal tract in Araçatuba/SP, found Strongyloides sp. in the stomach of capybaras and Capillaria hydrochoeri in the stomach and small intestine. These studies reinforce the findings of the genera Capillaria sp. and Strongyloides sp. in Maranhão and extend the area of occurrence of this genus in Brazil and in this host. As mentioned by Sinkoc et al. (2009) and Souza et al. (2021), cohabitation between domestic species and capybaras can favour the cycles of endoparasites in flooded environments, even accidentally. In the Trichuridae family, Petroneto et al. (2019) mention Trichuris vulpis in an equine in Espírito Santo, which cohabit pastures with cattle, and which are generally found parasitising the caecum and colon of domestic mammals (cattle, sheep, camels, pigs and dogs). Thus, efforts are being made to assess endoparasites simultaneously in different animal species cohabiting with capybaras, i.e. monitoring at the same time and in the same physical space (same biosystem). In the structure of the helminthic fauna in capybaras in Maranhão, Trichostrongylidae; Strongyloides sp, Capillaria sp and the protozoan Eimeria sp are similar to the results described in Acre in 2011, when Santos et al. evaluated parasite control in capybaras in a semi-extensive system, and in São Paulo in free-living capybaras, described by Santarém et al. (2006). In Argentina, Corriale et al., in 2011, cited Capillaria hydrochoeri, Strongyloides sp. and the Trichostrongyloidea family as nematodes, as well as Eimeria sp., among other findings in commercial capybaras.

Table 2 lists 15 articles published on endoparasites in South America, whether Platyhelminthes (flat worms) or Nematelminthes (cylindrical worms), found in capybaras in the natural environment in the South of the Americas. With several mentions of helminths from the Trichostrongyloidea superfamily since Travassos (1922), and mentions of Strongyloides sp. by Corriale et al. (2011) and Capillaria sp. by Jones (2021), further studies should be carried out to evaluate individuals and ecosystems throughout Brazil.

Table 2. Endoparasites found in capybaras in natural environments in South America (1922 to 2021).

Location	Species	Author
Brazil (MT)	Nudacotyle valdevaginatus, Neocotyle neocotyle, Taxorchis schistocotyle, Hippocrepis hippocrepis	Travassos (1922)
Brazil (RJ)	Nudacotyle tertius	Travassos (1939)
Venezuela	Vianella hydrochoeri, Capillaria hydrochoeri, Protozoophaga obesa, Dirofilaria acutiuscula, Monoecocestus decrescens, Hippocrepis hippocrepis, Taxorchis schistocotyle	Tarbes (1979)
Brazil (MS)	Vianella hydrochoeri, Hydrochoerisnema anomalobursata, Haemonchus sp., Trichostrongylus axei, Cooperia punctata, C. pectinata	Arantes (1983)
Bolivia	Vianella hydrochoeri, P. obesa, Habronema clarki, Monoecocestus hagmanni, M. macrobursatum, M. hydrochoeri, T. schistocotyle, H. hippocrepis	Casas et al. (1995)

Brazil (RS)	Strongyloides sp., C. hydrochoeri, V. hydrochoeri, H. anomalobursata, P. obesa, Trichuris spp., Monoecocestus jacobi, M. hydrochoeri, H. hippocrepis, T. schistocotyle, Neocladorchis cabrali	Sinkoc (1997)
Brazil (MS)	T. axei, V. hydrochoeri, H. anomalobursata, S. chapini, C. hydrochoeri, P. obesa, M. hagmanni, M. macrobursatum, M. hydrochoeri, Nudacotyle valdevaginatus, N. tertius, Neocotyle neocotyle, H. hippocrepis, T. schistocotyle	Bonutti (2002)
Venezuela	V. hydrochoeri, P. obesa, Monoecocestus macrobursatum, Monoecocestus hagmanni, H. hippocrepis, T. schistocotyle	Salas and Herrera (2004)
Brazil (SP)	Fasciola hepatica	Santarém et al. (2006)
Brazil (RS)	Capillaria hydrochoeri, Hydrochoerisnema anomalobursata, Protozoophaga obesa, Monoecocestus hagmanni, Monoecocestus macrobursatum, M. hagmanni and M. macrobursatum	Wendt (2009)
Brazil (AC)	Families: Trichostrongylidae; Strongyloididae (Strongyloides sp.); Trichuridae (Capillaria sp.)	Santos et al. (2011)
Argentina	Strongyloides sp.	Corriale et al. (2011)
Brazil (MG)	Trematoda: Notocotylidae - Hippocrepis hippocrepis	Assis et al. (2019)
Trinidad and Tobago	Trichuris spp.	Jones (2021)
Brazil (SP)	Classes Cestoda (Monoecocestus spp.), Digenea and Nematoda (Trichostrongyloidea, Strongyloides chapini, Protozoophaga obesa and Capillaria hydrochoeri) and Fasciola hepatica. Oocysts of the coccidia Eimeria spp. and Cryptosporidium spp.	Souza et al. (2021)

Wendt (2009), evaluating zooparasites in capybaras in a semi-intensive rearing system in the southern region of Rio Grande do Sul, found Capillaria hydrochoeri in adults and chicks. In the same year, he made older references to specimens found in Brazil and Venezuela, citing other authors and survey years (Table 2), such as Capillaria hydrochoeri, found by Tarbes (1979) in Venezuela, Trichostrongylus axei seen by Arantes (1983) in Mato Grosso do Sul, while Costa & Catto (1994) and Bonutti et al. (2002) saw T. axei, S. chapini, C.

hydrochoeri in the Pantanal-sul-matogrossense region and in Rio Grande do Sul they saw Strongyloides sp, C. hydrochoeri, Trichuris spp. in the citation by Sinkoc (1997). It is therefore possible that the Capillaria sp. in the Maranhão study is Capillaria hydrochoeri, but further studies are needed to confirm this. The Trichostrongylidae family, the Trichostrongyloidea superfamily, are small, slender nematodes with a vestigial or absent buccal capsule, and the males have a well-developed copulatory pouch. The Haemonchus and Ostertagia genera, which have a haematophagous habit, cause anaemia mainly in young animals and can produce submandibular oedema due to hypoalbuminaemia (MARTINS, 2019). Due to the polyparasitism found in the state, it is understood that there may be animals with low body scores, high morbidity and mortality, mainly in capybaras in Maranhão, without notification to the veterinary authorities, since it is not mandatory and further studies can elucidate the genera and species of the Trichostrongylidae family. The results of this research draw attention, as there is concern about mortality from trichostrongylosis, as there was an outbreak in Mato Grosso do Sul (2016), in a Nelore herd, where some adult cows died after showing weight loss, diarrhoea and remaining in decubitus. The recovery of helminths from the abomasum showed that Trichostrongylus axei was the main aetiological agent (LIMA et al. 2022). In addition to its presence in capybaras (ARANTES et al., 1983; BONUTI et al., 2002), the presence of Trichostrongylus axei is common in large and small ruminants (DA SILVA et al. 2018; LIMA et al. 2022), so these parasitic problems may be affecting capybaras in Maranhão.

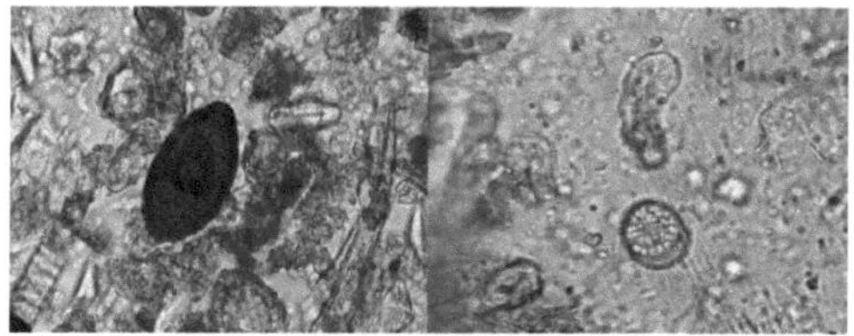

Figure 4 - On the left, an egg of Capillaria sp. and on the right, an oocyst of Coccidia sp. Photos: Chaves, 2021.

In the municipalities of Maranhão (table 3 and figure 5), the capybaras had two superfamilies of endoparasites, Trichostrongyloidea and Trichuroidea, the Stongyloididae family, as well as protozoa, so the capybaras were infected with an Eimeriidae family, and in the municipality of Balsas/MA, it was observed that one of the individuals, number 09, had diarrhoea due to pasty faeces. Eimeria ichiloensis and Eimeria trinidadensis have already been associated with diarrhoea in capybaras (JONES et al., 2019). In Balsas, in the cerrado biome, Eimeria sp. was evident in 43% of the samples. The high frequency of endoparasitism (100%) in the samples (table 3 and figure 5) raises the suspicion of morbidity and mortality from verminosis, especially in younger capybaras and during the dry season. This reinforces the need for further monitoring of capybara endoparasites in various biomes in Maranhão, for evaluation in dry and rainy periods, with observational analysis of clinical signs, body score (0 to 5), morbidity and mortality rates. In the Order Rodentia, Jones in 2021 carried out a review of Trichuris spp in neotropical rodents, citing its presence in Capybaras (Hydrochoerus hydrochaeris), Guinea Pigs (Cavia porcellus), Cutia (Dasyprocta leporina), and Paca (Agouti paca).

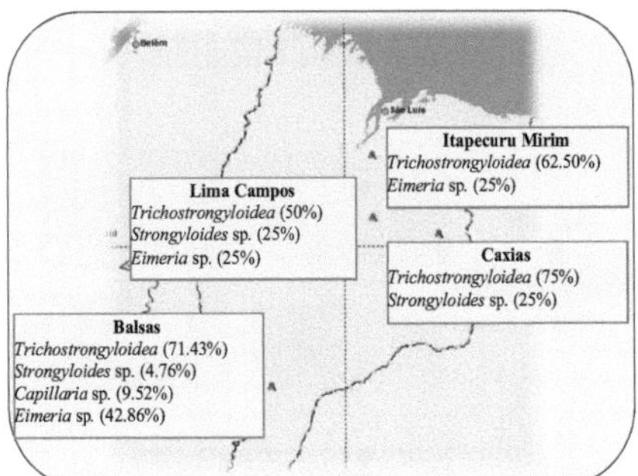

Figure 5: Locations of the collections indicated in red symbols in TrackMaker, with the respective percentages of parasites per municipality.

Among the zoonotic endoparasites, Cryptosporidium spp and Giardia spp were found in capybara droppings, due to exposure to untreated sewage in the soil of the Chico Mendes Municipal Natural Park/RJ (NORBERG et al., 2020). Therefore, it is interesting to carry out surveys in areas that have been anthropised due to their coexistence with capybaras and environmental contamination.

In São Paulo, Cryptosporidium spp oocysts were detected (SOUZA et al., 2021), as well as in Rio de Janeiro (NORBERG et al., 2020) and Espírito Santo, Fasciola hepatica (MARTINS et al., 2021). Thus, further monitoring of the biosystems inhabited by capybaras in Maranhão and the detection of zoonotic endoparasites in new surveys are expected. The municipality of Balsas in Maranhão stands out for its wealth of endoparasites in 21 samples, either due to the presence of helminths from the Trichostrongyloidea superfamily (71 per cent), Capillaria sp. (92%), Strongyloides sp (5%) or the oocysts of protozoa, Eimeria sp (43%) in capybaras, with the light blue colour highlighting the visualisation of the data analysed in the presentation, displayed in insights in the Power BI panel blocks (figure 6).

Figure 6. Distribution of helminths and protozoa in capybaras in the 4 municipalities of Maranhão.

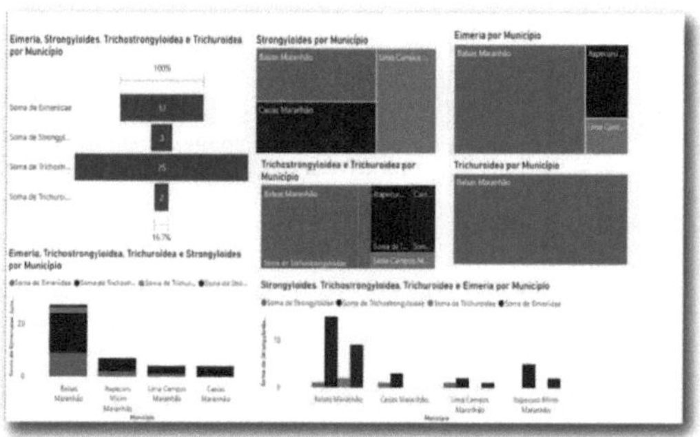

Source: Microsoft Power BI Desktop. Version: 2.122.746.0 64-bit (Oct 2023)

In Colombia, in a public health approach, two zoonotic parasites, Plagorchis muris and Neobalantidium coli, have been identified circulating in wild synanthropic capybaras, thus, they considered that it is very important to expand ecoepidemiological studies to other wildlife species, as it will contribute to early detection and prevention of parasitic repercussion events within the One Health concept (URIBE, et al., 2021). The striped field mouse (Apodemus agrarius) is a natural and definitive host for Plagorchis muris, and infection rates and parasite loads vary seasonally and geographically in South Korea (CHAI et al., 2007).
Cattle and capybaras are thought to share the same feeding, resting and watering areas in various parts of South and Central America. In Colombia, Giraldo-Forero & Murcia-Martínez (2019) surveyed the prevalence of zoonotic gastrointestinal parasites in a beef slaughterhouse plant in the municipality of Fómeque-Cundinamarca, highlighting the presence of protozoa and helminths, namely: Neobalantidium coli, Strongyloides spp and Fasciola hepatica, which by their nature are zoonotic agents. Neobalantidium coli has been found in pigs and wild boar (Sus scrofa) in Iran, as well as in pigs in Venezuela (NOORPISHEH GHADIMI et al., 2014; VALLES, 2021). These new zoonotic endoparasites are therefore worth investigating in new state surveys of large and small wild rodents, such as the cattle and pigs mentioned above, due to their spatial and temporal coexistence. Gastrointestinal nematode infections in pigs and especially poultry are thought to be on the rise due to new methods of free-range farming (DISCONTOOLS, 2023). As capybaras live freely in rural and wild environments, they have high parasitism and acquired resistance. OJASTI (2009) cites that the capybara is a remnant of giant rodents that evolved in South America during the last 10 million years.Coccidiosis is known to cause lesions in the digestive tract of animals and economic losses on farms (FITZGERALD, 1980). Some pathogens can clinically cause bloody diarrhoea with fibrin (BUSATO et al., 1998). The capybaras observed during the collections in Maranhão were in good body condition and there were no clinical signs compatible with parasitic diseases caused by Eimeria sp.Rodríguez-Durán and

collaborators (2015), investigating protozoa (in summer and winter) in wild capybaras in Colombia, mention that mothers and their young are more likely to be infected among the susceptible groups, and it was more evident that in the dry season there was greater parasitism. They claim that Eimeria sp. in the period of their study, did not register a significant increase, possibly due to the need to sporulate with oxygen at high temperatures (27 °C) and high environmental humidity (>80%). Albuquerque et al. (2008) reported several species of Eimeria in Brazil, Bolivia and Venezuela, namely E. trinidadensis, E. ichiloensis, E. boliviensis, E. araside, E. capibarae and E. hidrochoeri.
Historically, Eimeria capibarae and Eimeria hydrochoeri were reported by Carini in 1937, but there are few references of these protozoa in capybaras in South America and nothing in Central America (Table 4). Further research in Maranhão should be carried out on capybara faeces in order to identify genera and species related to coexisting herbivores, as well as to identify other parasites with zoonotic potential.

Table 3. Detection of protozoan infection in capybaras in South America.

Location	Species	Author
Brazil (SP)	Eimeria capibarae, E. hydrochoeri	Carini (1937)
Venezuela	Eimeria capibarae, Eimeria hydrochaeris	Ruiz and Rivera (1981)
Bolivia, Venezuela	Eimeria trinidadensis, Eimeria ichiloensis, Eimeria boliviensis	Casas, Duszynski and Zalles (1995)
Argentina	Eimeria spp.	Martínez et al. (1998)
Venezuela	Eimeria spp.	Moreno et al. (1999)
Argentina	Eimeria sp.	Ortiz and Rizzello (2004)
Argentina	Eimeria sp.	Santa Cruz et al. (2005)
Brazil (RS)	Eimeria ichiloensis, E.trinidadensis, E.boliviensis, Eimeria sp.	Gurgel (2005)
Brazil (RS)	Eimeria araside	Gurgel, Sartori and Araújo (2007)
Brazil (BA)	Eimeria trinidadensis, E. ichiloensis	Albuquerque et al. (2008)
Brazil (RS)	Eimeria ichiloensis	Silva et al. (2007)
Brazil (RS)	Eimeria sp.	Reginatto et al. (2008)

Figure 7 and Figure 8 show the good body scores of the free-living capybaras, which were captured on a property in Santa Inês/MA.

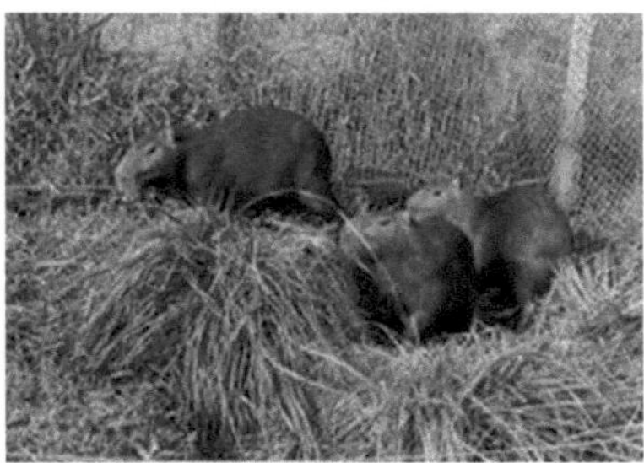

Figure 7. Free-living capybaras captured on a property in Santa Inês/MA

It should also be noted that capybaras are bioindicators for demonstrating parasite dispersal routes to subpopulations, be they other rodents or domestic animals, since they cohabit in humid environments, share contaminated water and graze together, so they should be constantly monitored, considering parasitic zoonoses and/or the spread of parasites to animals.

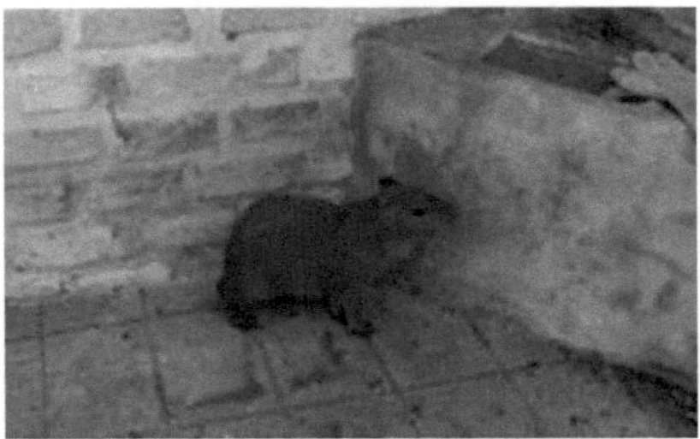

Figure 8. Male capybara cub, approximately 3 months old, caught on a property in Santa Inês/MA.

In evaluating the coexistence of capybaras, domestic herbivores in rural areas of Maranhão, whether with angulates and/or solipeds, it is understood that in the case of eimeriosis and verminoses, new studies should be carried out on various coexisting species, specifying the genera and species of the endoparasites, in order to be more specific in inferring interactions in the ecosystem, as well, The studies will give us the opportunity to lower production costs with deworming and/or therapeutic treatments, as well as providing us with opportunities to establish satisfactory prophylactic measures, such as avoiding contact with wildlife through fences, pasture rotation taking into account parasite cycles, in order to reduce economic losses on farms. In this way, the study emphasises the importance of veterinarians, among other agricultural professionals, in the theme of 'one health', thus considering the biological cycles of parasites, biosystems, pathology in hosts and the zoonotic potential of a species in a synanthropic character and the spillover between species.

CONCLUSION

This study reveals that capybaras have helminths from the Trichostrongyloidea and Trichuroidea superfamilies (Capillaria sp.) and Strongyloididae family (Strongyloides sp.) and Eimeria sp. oocysts, as well as their pathogenic potential due to their interrelationship in 'single health', in the environment, where domestic animals, wild animals and man himself cohabit, whether in peri-urban and/or rural areas.

REFERENCES

ALBUQUERQUE, G. R. et al. Eimerid coccidia from capybaras (Hydrochoerus hydrochaeris) in southern Bahia, Brazil. **Pesquisa Veterinária Brasileira,** v. 28, n. 7, p. 323-328, 2008.

ALVES, L. F. S. et al. Literature review on cecotrophagy in capybaras (Hydrochaeris hydrochaeris). VI SIMPÓSIO DE CIÊNCIAS DA UNESP - Dracena. Faculty of Agricultural Sciences, Federal University of Grande Dourados (UFGD), Dourados, **Proceedings**, 2010. 3p.

AMARANTE, Alessandro Francisco Talamini do; RAGOZO, Alessandra; SILVA, Bruna Fernanda da. Sheep parasites. 2014. 254p. Available at https://static.scielo.org/scielobooks/nv4nc/pdf/amarante-9788568334423.pdf

ASSIS, J. C. A. et al. A morphological, molecular and life cycle study of the capybara parasite Hippocrepis hippocrepis (Trematoda: Notocotylidae). **Plos One**, v. 14, n. 8, e0221662, 2019.

BASSAN, Lucas Maciel, et al. "Strongylosis: literature review." **CientÍfica Eletrônica de Medicina Veterinária**, São Paulo 11.6 (2008): 1-7.

BONUTI, M. R. et al. Gastrointestinal helminths of capybaras (Hydrochoerus hydrochaeris) in the Paiaguás sub-region, Pantanal of Mato Grosso do Sul, Brazil. **Semina: Ciências Agrárias**, Londrina, v. 23, n. 1, p. 57-62, 2002.

BUSATO A. et al. A case control study of potential enteric pathogens for calves raised in cow-calf herds. **Journal Veterinary Medicine,** n. 45, p. 519-528, 1998.

CHAI, J. Y., Park, J. H., Guk, S. M., Kim, J. L., Kim, H. J., Kim, W. H., ... & Baek, L. J. (2007). Plagiorchis muris infection in Apodemus agrarius from northern Gyeonggi-do (Province) near the demilitarised zone. The Korean journal of parasitology, 45(2), 153.

CORRIALE, M. J. et al. Prevalence of gastrointestinal parasites in a natural population of capybaras, Hydrochoerus hydrochaeris, in Esteros del Iberá (Argentina). **Ibero-Latin American Journal of Parasitology,** v. 70, n. 2, p. 189-196, 2011.

COSTA, C.A.F. & CATTO, J.B. Helminth parasites of capybaras (Hydrochaeris hydrochaeris) in the Nhecolândia sub-region, Pantanal-sul-matogrossense. Rev. Bras. Biol., v.51, n.1, p.39- 48, 1994.

COSTA, D. S. et al. Capybara Reproduction. **Arquivos de Ciências Veterinária e Zoologia UNIPAR**, n. 5, p. 111-118, 2002.

CUETO, G. R. Diseases of Capybara. In MOREIRA JR, FERRAZ KMPMB, HERRERA
EA, MACDONALD DW. **Capybara. Biology, Use and Conservation of an Exceptional Neotropical Species.** Springer. New York, 2013, Chapter 9, 160-184p.

DA SILVA ROBERTO, Francisca Fernanda et al. Gastrointestinal nematodes in beef sheep farming under grazing regime. **Pubvet**, v. 12, p. 147, 2018.

DISCONTOOLS PROJECT MANAGER. **About us.** 2023. Available at https://www.discontools.eu/about.html.

FARIKOSKI, IO., Medeiros, LS., Carvalho, YK., Ashford, DA., Figueiredo, EES., Fernandes, DVGS., Silva, PJB., & Ribeiro, VMF. (2019). The urban and rural capybaras (Hydrochoerus hydrochaeris)
as reservoir of Salmonella in the western Amazon, Brazil. **Brazilian Veterinary Research,** 39 (1), 66-69.

FITZGERALD P. R. The economic impact of coccidiosis in domestic animals. **Advances Veterinary Science Comparative Medicine,** n. 4, p. 121-143, 1980

FONTANA, I. **Evaluating the role of the Montiro pig in the chain Epidemiological analysis of leptospirosis in sub-regions of the Pantanal of Mato Grosso do Sul.** (Master's thesis). Faculty of Agronomy and Veterinary Medicine, University of Brasilia. 2011. 61 p

FORERO-MONTAÑA, J.; BETANCUR, J.; CAVELIER, J. Hydrochaeris (Rodentia: Hydrochaeridae) in Caño Limón, Arauca, Colombia. **Article in Revista de Biologia Tropical,** v.51, n. 2, p. 579-589, 2003.

GIRALDO-FORERO, J. C., & Murcia-Martínez, X. J. (2019). Estudio piloto de frecuencia de parásitos gastrointestinales zoonóticos en bovinos sacrificados en la planta de beneficio del municipio de Fómeque Cundinamarca-Colombia en el primer semestre del 2018.

GONZÁLEZ-Jiménez, E. 1995. **The capibara. Current state of its**

production. FAO. Rome. Serie Estudio Producción y Sanidad Animal, 122. 112 pp.

HERRERA, E. A. Growth and dispersal of capybaras, Hydrochaeris hydrochaeris, in the llanos of Venezuela. **Journal Zoologia (London)**, n. 228, p. 307-316, 1992.

HOSKEN, F.M.; SILVEIRA, A. C. 2002. **Capybara breeding**. UFV. Viçosa/MG. 298p.

JONES, Kegan Romelle; LALL, Kavita Ranjeeta; GARCIA, Gary Wayne. Endoparasites of selected native non-domesticated mammals in the neotropics (New World Tropics). **Veterinary sciences**, v. 6, n. 4, p. 87, 2019.

JONES, K R. Trichuris spp. in Animals, with Specific Reference to Neo-Tropical Rodents.**Veterinary Science,** v. 8, n. 2, p. 15, 2021.

LIGNON JS, Soares Martins N, Mueller A, et al. **Prevalence of intestinal nematodes in draught horses in the city of Pelotas/RS, Brazil.** RVZ. 18 July 2020; 27:1-6. Available at: https://rvz.emnuvens.com.br/rvz/article/view/439

LIMA, Stephanie C. et al. Mortality caused by gastrointestinal nematodes in beef cattle submitted to inadequate sanitary protocol. **Pesquisa Veterinária Brasileira**, v. 42, 2022.

MACDONALD, D. W. Dwindling resources and the social behaviour of capybaras (Hydrochoerus hydrochaeris) (Mammalia). **Journal Zoology (London),** n. 194, p. 371-391, 1981.

MARTINS, Isabella Vilhena Freire. **Veterinary parasitology.** EDUFES. Vitória - ES, 2. ed. 2019. 320 p. Available at https://repositorio.ufes.br/bitstream/10/11421/1/parasitologia-veterinaria_livro-digital.pdf

MARTINS, Isabella Vilhena Freire et al. Molecular confirmation of Fasciola hepatica infection in capybaras (Hydrochoerus hydrochaeris) from the State of

Espírito Santo, Brazil. **Brazilian Journal of Veterinary Parasitology**, v. 30, 2021.

MENDES, A. et al. A note on the cecotrophy behaviour in capybara (Hydrochaeris hydrochaeris).

Applied Animal Behaviour Science, n. 66, p. 161-167, 2000.

MERKER BREYER, Gabriela et al. Wild capybaras as reservoir of shiga toxin-producing Escherichia coli in urban Amazonian Region. **Letters in Applied Microbiology,** v. 75, n. 1, p. 10-16, 2022.

MONES, A.; MARTINEZ, S. Estudios sobre la familia Hydrochoeridae (Rodentia) XIII. Parasitosis and pathologies of Hydrochoerus Brisson, 1972. **Revista de la facultad de humanidades y** Ciencias, Serie Ciencias Biológicas, n. 1, p. 297-329, 1982.

MOREIRA, J. R. et al. **Capybara. Biology, Use and Conservation of an Exceptional Neotropical Species**. Springer. New York, 2013. 424p.

MOURÃO, Nadja Maria. Amazônia Maranhense, Cerrado and Communities: the "look" of design on the environmental context. 2022.

NORBERG, Antonio Neres et al. Cryptosporidium spp. Oocysts and Giardia spp. cysts in faeces of Capybaras (Hydrochoerus hydrochaeris) from Chico Mendes Natural Municipal Park, city of Rio de Janeiro, Brazil: **potential risk for zoonotic transmission.** 2020.

NOGUEIRA MF. CRUZ TF. Capybara diseases. Corumbá, MS: Embrapa Pantanal, 2007. 74 p.
https://www.alice.cnptia.embrapa.br/bitstream/doc/805195/1/Livro030.pdf

NOORPISHEH GHADIMI, Shamsi et al. Neobalantidium coli: first molecular identification from the Eurasian wild boar, Sus scrofa in Bushehr province, southwestern Iran. **Veterinary Medicine and Science,** v. 6, n. 1, p. 142-146, 2020.

OJASTI, J. The capybara, its biology and management. **Tropical Biology and**

Conservation Management, v. 10, p. 323-340, 2009.

PETRONETO, BS. Callegari, BF. Poncio AC. et al. Trichuris vulpis (Nematoda: Trichuridae) in a horse (Equus caballus): case report. In book: Studies in Veterinary Medicine 2. April 2019. DOI: 10.22533/at.ed.7081916046

RAMOS, Fernanda Gomes Castelan. Parasites of domestic mammals in the Serra da Capivara National Park, southeast Piauí-Brazil. 2011. 107 f. Master's thesis. **Sergio Arouca National School of Public Health**, Rio de Janeiro, 2011.

RODRÍGUEZ-DURÁN, A.; PALMA, L. C. B.; FLÓREZ, R. P. Principales protozoarios gastrointestinales en chigüiros silvestres (Hydrochoerus hydrochaeris) en una vereda del municipio de Arauca, Colombia. **Zootecnia Tropical**, v. 33, n. 3, p. 261-268, 2015.

SANTARÉM, V. A. et al. Fasciola hepatica in capybara. **Acta Tropica**. v. 98, p. 311-313. 2006.

SANTOS, F. G. A. et al. Control of intestinal parasites in capybaras (Hydrochaerus hydrachaeris) raised in a semi-extensive system in the municipality of Senador Guimard Santos, Acre. **Acta Veterinária Brasílica**, v.5, n.4, p.393-398, 2011.

SHIMABUKURO, Juliana Suieko. Study of the seroprevalence of Leptospira spp. in capybaras (Hydrochaeris hydrochaeris) in the Alto Tietê catchment area, SP. 2006. Master's thesis, University of São Paulo, São Paulo, SP, Brazil. 2006.

SILVA, Jefferson Noronha Bezerra, et al. "Pharmacological treatment of strongyloidiasis in humans: an integrative review." **Revista de Medicina** 102.5 (2023).

SINKOC A.L. Brum F.A. Muller G. Brum J.G.W. Helminth parasites of capybara (Hydrochoerus hydrochaeris L. 1766) in the Araçatuba region, São Paulo, Brazil. Arq. Inst. Biol., São Paulo, v.71, n.3, p.329-333, jul./set., 2004

SOUZA, S. L. P. et al. Endoparasites of capybaras (Hydrochoerus hydrochaeris) from anthropised and natural areas of Brazil. **Revista Brasileira de**

Parasitologia Veterinária, n. 30, v. 2, 2021.

VIEIRA, F. M.; LIMA, S. S.; DE A. BESSA, E. C. Morphology and biometry of eggs and larvae of Strongyloides sp. Grassi, 1879 (Rhabditoidea: Strongyloididae) gastrointestinal parasite of Hydrochaeris hydrochaeris (Linnaeus, 1766) (Rodentia: Hydrochaeridae), in the municipality of Juiz de Fora, Minas Gerais. **Revista Brasileira de Parasitologia Veterinária,** v. 15, n. 1, p. 7- 12, 2006.

URIBE, M., Hermosilla, C., Rodríguez-Durán, A., Vélez, J., López-Osorio, S., Chaparro- Gutiérrez, J. J., & Cortés-Vecino, J. A. (2021). Parasites circulating in wild synanthropic capybaras (Hydrochoerus hydrochaeris): a one health approach. Pathogens, 10(9), 1152

VALLES, Luis Eduardo Traviezo. Balantidium nawaraoi n. sp., in the Warao community of Nabasanuka, Venezuela. Revista Médica Sinergia, v. 6, n. 02, p. 1-11, 2021.

WENDT, Luciana Welter. **Parasitic fauna of capybaras** (Hydrochoerus hydrochaeris Linnaeus, 1766) **in a semi-intensive breeding system in the southern region of Rio Grande do Sul**. 2009. Master's dissertation. Federal University of Pelotas. Pelotas, 2009. 52f.

WILLIS, H. H. A simple levitation method for the detection of hookworm ova. **The Medical Journal of Australia**, v. 2, n. 18, p. 375-376, 1921

CHAPTER II

CAPYBARAS IN MARANHÃO: A GUIDE FOR EDUCATIONAL PURPOSES AND PRESERVATION OR CONTROL

Roberto C. N. de Arruda, Helder de Moraes Pereira, Viviane Correia Silva Coimbra, Hamilton Pereira Santos, Francisco Borges Costa, Hermes Ribeiro Luz

PRESENTATION

The main focus of the book "Capivaras no Maranhão: Guia orientativa para fins educativos, de preservação ou controle" is to describe the behavioural characteristics and diseases of capybaras, as a way of understanding and preserving this wonderful animal. Capybaras are the largest rodents in the world and because of their natural habit of staying in bodies of water (dams, reservoirs, lakes, lagoons, rivers and streams), they are named after the genus Hydrochoerus, which is a reference to a water pig. They come from the genealogy of other American rodents, such as the prey, mocó, paca, agouti and others from the Caviidae family. In Tupi-Guarani "kapibara" means "grass eater", these animals live in flooded areas or firm areas with water, in Brazil, only they don't inhabit the caatinga biome.Semi-aquatic, they have membranes between the toes of their forelimbs and hind limbs that make swimming easier. They usually live well with domestic animals on farms, wild animals in rural areas or in the wild. They tend to be docile, but in areas close to urban environments, if they feel cornered, they can attack humans, dogs or other pets. In the wild, they can live up to twelve years.Their natural environment is being degraded and they are moving closer to humans. Normally, they move around constantly in search of places with water and food (an average of 3 to 5 kilometres in this dispersal). However, they are generally undemanding and their herds are growing close to aquatic environments in various municipalities in the state. Their predators in Maranhão are disappearing; previously they were easily found with jaguars, alligators and anacondas. They use bodies of water to protect themselves from attacks by carnivores and humans and can stay underwater for more than five minutes. The abundance of water helps them to lose heat, reproduce and avoid contact with predators.

The species lives in a closed society, with a dominant male, a group of females and cubs, so there are around 20 to 30 animals, but they can be found in smaller or larger groups. The males fight over territories and females, and the subordinate males, who are not expelled from the flock, remain and help with surveillance by making a warning click or bark when dangers are detected. With high reproductive competence due to its fertility and fecundity, it has a high potential to have two pregnancies a year, with an average of 4 offspring per birth, and a good survival rate for the young.

Sometimes these animals are found eating their own faeces, which is common in rabbits, hares and other rodents, i.e. a natural and adapted way of digesting fibres and nutrients that would otherwise be eliminated, but it could also be favourable for maintaining some types of infections and/or internal parasitism.

Finally, this book is aimed at students and professionals in environmental and agricultural science careers, as another bibliographic source of reference on the subject.

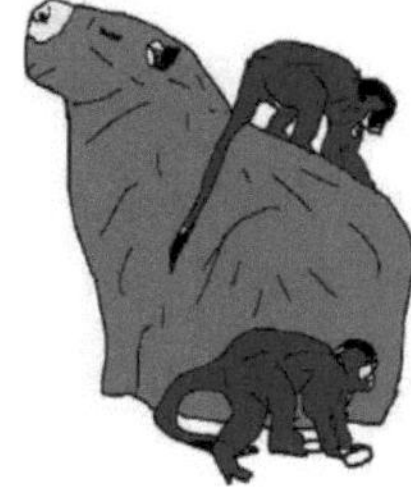

FEATURES

They are hardy, gregarious, free-living mammals and herbivores, and represent the largest known rodent in the world, in Tupi-Guarani "kapibara" means "grass eater". Females weigh an average of 50kg and males 60kg. Depending on their environment, they measure between 1.0 and 1.30 m in length and 0.50 to 0.60 m in height. However, specimens weighing more than 100 kg live weight (kg/LW) have been reported in anthropised environments. At birth, the cub weighs approximately 2 kg, while weaning takes place between 8 and 12 weeks at 5 to 15 kg/PV.They are semi-aquatic animals, with four (04) digits on their forelimbs and three (03) on the back. The interdigital spaces are joined by a membrane which facilitates swimming, long dives and big dives. With the curvature of the spine, the body has a rounder shape. The limbs are short in relation to the body. The head is large and the muzzle wide, with a voluminous, short neck. Their coat varies from reddish-brown to grey, and their genitals are hidden (protected) in an anal sac and have no tail. Their upper lip has slits similar to those of rabbits, and their eyes are large and developed for night vision. When they are swimming, they balance their heads above water, and the position of their eyes, ears and nostrils make it easier for them to observe and see the external environment when swimming. The incisor teeth of adults are between 5 and 7 cm long and need to be worn down on a daily basis, or broken off spontaneously; if natural wear did not occur, it could cause injuries to the animals' mouths.

HABITAT AND BEHAVIOUR

They live in groups with an alpha (dominant) male, multiple females, young individuals and beta (subordinate) males. The alpha male is significantly heavier than the subordinates, so to preserve the species, the males, betas or satellites, are not expelled from the group and serve to warn of dangers with high-frequency calls, such as a bark. They also use whistles, cackles, teeth chattering and clicks to communicate.

Native to the American continent, they live for up to 12 years on the banks of rivers, dams and lakes in family groups, and use water for all vital activities, such as reproduction and protection. They can be found from South to Central America, more specifically from northern Argentina to Panama, preferably in areas with an abundance of water. They are not seen in the arid areas of Brazil, such as the northeastern caatinga, and in South America, they are absent in Chile.

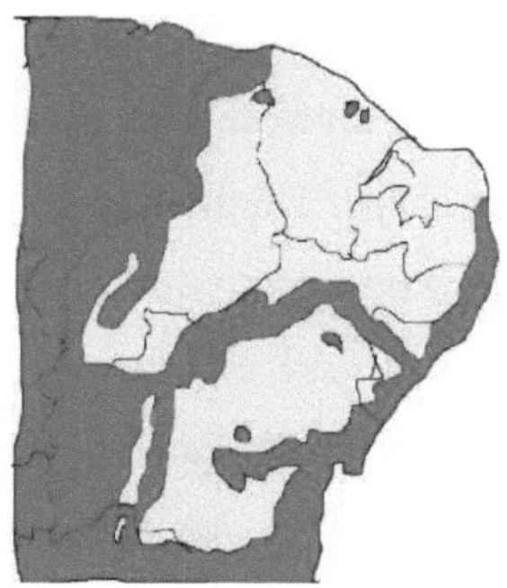

Due to its evolution in the aquatic environment and its digestive system from a herbivore, the capybara eats grasses in particular, but enjoys grazing near water in natural environments. They also inhabit savannahs, woodlands, mangroves, wet and dry forests, and if their diet is limited, they travel between areas for 3 to 5 kilometres. On the trails or paths, faeces can be found in the form of syllables or acorns and footprints, due to the fact that they almost always move in single file.They use the water as shelter from predatory carnivores, as they can stay submerged for more than five (5) minutes. With deforestation and plantations, some of their predators (jaguars, caimans, snakes or wild carnivores) are diminishing, with the exception of man as a hunter.In areas where there is a high density of individuals, they can compete with livestock for fodder, or even invade and destroy crops, as well as deteriorating the quality of water supplied to domestic animals, or even becoming synanthropic.We must also consider the wide-ranging negative consequences of the degradation of their habitat, as their continued existence in natural environments requires favourable agriculture and the preservation of biomes. It is therefore important to conserve capybaras in their natural environment and prevent them from living with humans and spreading diseases.

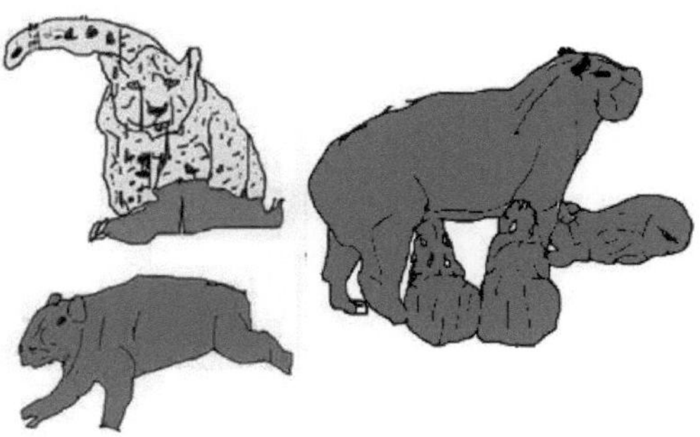

It was observed that the animals move around the rivers and streams in the interior of Maranhão, depending on the availability of food. Thus, their location alternates over the course of the year or dry or rainy climate cycles.

A unique act of capybaras is eating soft faeces, which consists of ingesting a specific type of excrement produced in the caecum (cecotrophs) extracted from the end of the rectum. This has been widely observed in rabbits and hares, which are from the lagomorph family, but it also occurs in other rodents. The differences between these two families is that lagomorphs have 02 pairs of upper incisor teeth and 01 pair of lower incisor teeth (06 teeth), while rodents have 04 incisor teeth.

The capybara has good fertility and fecundity, and in the state of Maranhão, the number of individuals has been increasing, as we have few natural predators in the food chain, and good pasture conditions in the rainy season, so naturally there are interactions with domestic and wild animals, as well as in the dry season, there is a shortage of pasture and food, bringing proximity between the various species in the same environment.

REPRODUCTION

The capybara is one of the most fertile and fecund herbivores. The adult male is characterised by a glandular protuberance on the upper part of the snout, which is oval-shaped and hairless, and is actually made up of a cluster of sebaceous glands that expel pheromones. Males reach sexual maturity at over 12 months of age, weighing an average of 30 to 40kg.

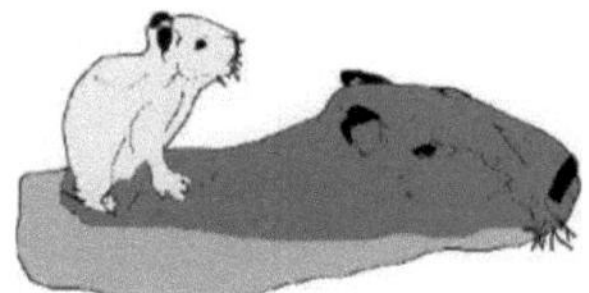

A fold of skin covers the genitals and anus, giving the animal the appearance of a cloaca, so the testicles are not in a scrotum and can only be palpated through the abdomen.Females in the reproductive period have six pairs of teats and tend to breed all year round. They are sexually active and fertile from 01 (one) to 07 (seven) years of age, and these females are more gregarious.

Male betas occasionally form other subgroups with females and sometimes head off in other directions in search of pastures and breeding opportunities. Copulation takes place mainly in the water and occasionally on land. The male is capable of making up to 10 mounts in one hour (oestrus lasts less than 24 hours). The female's gestation period is approximately 150 days, and the number of cubs ranges from 1 to 8. There can be up to two (02) births a year, with an average of 4 cubs per birth and a high rate of weaned cubs. The birth period can occur during the rainy months in some areas and at birth the young weigh around 2kg. Mortality in adults is less than 1% under normal conditions, but predation and mortality are higher in infants, at around 15%. The behaviour of feeding offspring that are not their own favours synchronisation of the females' reproductive cycles, and in the wild, they seek out forests to give birth more peacefully.

ILLNESS

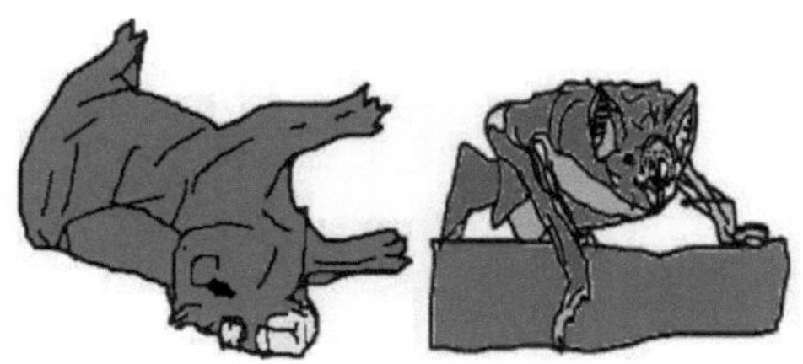

Capybaras have been hunted for their red meat and low-cholesterol fat, and for their hides. There is evidence that since pre-Columbian times (before the arrival of Europeans), they were an essential part of the diet of indigenous communities. Therefore, coexistence with humans and the consumption of meat are considered important from the point of view of public health, as well as being important for the coexistence and health of the animals.

Capybaras are infested by ticks of the genus Amblyomma (A. dubitatum, A. aureolatum, A. ovale and Amblyomma sculptum). ovale and Amblyomma sculptum) and the latter is the main vector and reservoir of the bacterium Rickettsia rickettsii, which causes Brazilian Spotted Fever (BSF) in the southeast of Brazil. However, in the state of Maranhão this disease has not yet been confirmed, and Amblyomma cajennense (sensu stricto) is the main species parasitising capybaras, but has not been associated with BSF.

Q fever has already been reported in French Guiana, so a survey was carried out in our state using the fresh faeces of some individuals, but the molecular PCR technique did not find the agent of this disease, the bacterium Coxiella burnetti.

In 2014 and 2020, capybaras were shown to have antibodies against Orthopoxvirus, so they could be the link between the wild and the urban environment in the viral maintenance of animal and bovine pox. In Maranhão, through PCR tests on faeces and blood, has not yet been detected.

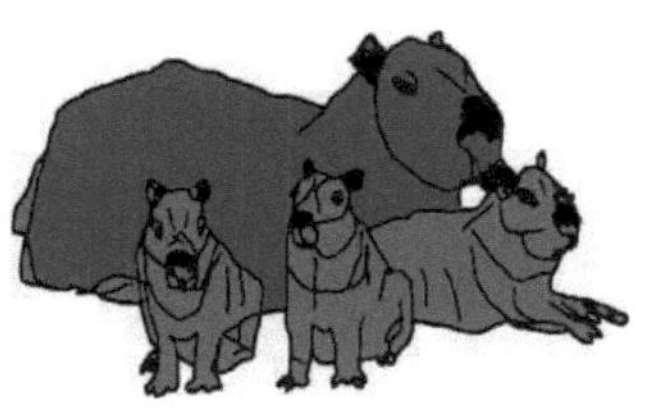

In Anchieta/SP in 2020, 03 (three) capybaras were killed by the rabies virus transmitted by the bat, Desmodus rotundus, the so-called 'desmodine rabies', as a result of the death of domestic animals and the removal of other herbivores from the area.Reports of sudden death, stress in captivity and septicaemia caused by Salmonella sp have already occurred in Botucatu/SP, as well as in urban and rural areas in the west of the Amazon.Capybaras were identified as reservoirs of Leptospira spp in Pernambuco, as well as in Maranhão in 2021. The first description of brucellosis in capybaras was in Argentina, where Brucella melitensis was isolated. In Maranhão, antibodies against Brucella abortus were not found in capybaras. A long time ago, two capybaras imported into a zoo in Germany, after coughing and losing weight, were diagnosed with tuberculosis and Mycobacterium bovis was isolated. In free-living capybaras in São Paulo, bacteria such as Escherichia coli 19 have already been isolated in the faeces, and coproparasitological analyses have also revealed parasites such as Protozoophaga sp., Strongyloides sp, Viannella spp, and eggs and larvae of Ancylostomidae. In the state of Maranhão, intestinal parasites from the Trichostrongyloidea Superfamily, Trichuroidea, (Capillaria sp. eggs) and Capillaria sp. family have been detected. Strongyloididae (eggs of Strongyloides sp.), and protozoa (Eimeria sp.), the star tick (Amblyomma cajennense sensu stricto) was also observed in the Amazon environment. There have been reports of Fasciola hepatica in RS, SC, SP and MG, outbreaks causing high mortality rates in capybaras, but there have been no reports in the state of Maranhão. Trypanosoma sp. has already been found in free-living capybaras in the Federal District, indicating that they could be vectors for trypanosomatid species.

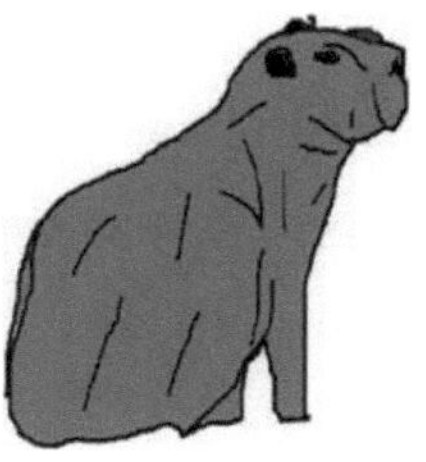

ECOLOGICAL CONTROL

Control can be carried out because of the potential economic risk to farm animals, or even because it may be a synanthropic species, due to public health, mainly because of R. rickettsii and the occurrence of FMB. Ecological control is the opposite of surgical reproductive control, be it vasectomy (deferentectomy) or tubal ligation (tubal ligation), and is the ecological control recommended by ESALQ/USP, which determines the mapping of capybara trails through footprints, faeces and the presence of star ticks. Areas with crops or pastures should be fenced off with fences (1.70 metre mesh and 2.5 inch mesh) and lines of underground tubular passageways (capivarodutos), to separate wild environments from watering holes, in order to avoid contact or coexistence with people and/or domestic animals, or even being run over. Non-lethal electric fences can be used on 3 wires or more, avoiding contact with woods or plants, as they steal current.

CAPYBARA MANAGEMENT IN CAPTIVITY

According to Nogueira Filho (2023) and Cleber Alho (1986), it is possible to contribute to the conservation, preservation or control of the species by treating them in an intensive system on small properties in a sustainable way, for the purpose of producing leather and meat with a low fat content, achieving good market prices for a specific and more capitalised consumer demand. Nogueira

Filho (2023) recommends that in intensive management, preference should be given to family groups, and gives the example of using 1 male to 8 females, in an area of 350 to 400 m^2 , with good watering in a pond that can be 20 m^2 (4 x 5 m), or taking advantage of a pond, puddle or lake that already exists on the property.

Roofs made of tiles or thatch should be up to 1.5 metres high over an area of at least 40 $metres^2$ in length, or even have tree or shrub shelters available for resting.

EMBRAPA recommends semi-extensive rearing, where the density can reach up to 5 capybaras per hectare, with the presence of dams or ponds, pasture without competition from cattle and horses, and a patch of woodland for resting and calving. Generally, they consider properties between 10 and 50 hectares in size, i.e. ranches or farms.

Capybaras feed on aquatic plants, weeds such as elephant grass and graze on grasses. They also adapt to leftover crops and grains, or by-products of rice, beans, soya, maize, millet and sugar cane. In Venezuela, captive animals were fed pig feed with 15 per cent crude protein.

Capybaras consume an average of 40 litres/animal/day, hence the need for good quality water in a float trough, while food should be in more than one trough, at a rate of 500g for pregnant females and 200 to 300g/day for other categories, remember that when starting treatment, you should adapt for 15 days, with half the final supply.

In Brazil, EMBRAPA researcher Pinheiro (2007) mentions the intensive regime, sexually mature females at around 10 to 12 months, producing 3 to 4 offspring/parturition, and having a birth weight of over 2kg, and he also mentions that mortality up to weaning was around 30.0 % and up to one year 15.0 %. The animals were slaughtered at 30kg at 12 months, with a carcass yield of 50 to 60 per cent.When considering breeding projects, the ideal is separation by category, or a group of 1 male to 5 to 8 females separated by paddocks; in other areas, you should calculate 20 m^2 /animal until completion in one year.

We recommend fences with wire mesh (12-gauge wire 1 metre high) and 2.5" mesh and smooth wire up to 1.5 metres high to contain the animals. These animals are very strong. There needs to be another area for quarantining sick or newly arrived animals of 50 to 100 metres^2 , or even calving paddocks of 10 metres .^{2}

Weanlings between 02 and 03 months old can be housed in 25 metre pens^2 , and should remain there until they reach slaughter weight of around 30kg.

According to Cleber Alho, a researcher at EMBRAPA (1986), Trypanosoma evansi can cause obstacles to the captive breeding system and he advises that every six months they should be given a polyvalent anthelmintic treatment, such as those used for cattle and horses, either orally with a bovine applicator, in mineral salt or food according to their live weight, and 1% ivermectin subcutaneously for worms, ticks and/or mange. We recommend checking daily for cases of myiasis and coccidiosis (or eimeriosis), which are common.

In Acre, it is generally recommended to deworm 6 times a year, every 2 months for adults, every 1 week after birth for young and once a month after that. Using oxfendazole orally as the active ingredient and Levamisole hydrochloride as an injection.Biosecurity in breeding is an investment in health, keeping breeding sites clean at all times, with waste removed, and equipment, clean clothes and footwear disinfected, as well as avoiding contact with rats, flies, birds or domestic animals (or even wild animals), keeping control of access by people and vehicles, as they can bring in microorganisms from other areas, in another line of thought, providing us with traceability of origin.

As a species of economic interest, there are materials in scientific literature and adjustments to procedures to comply with environmental legislation.

FINAL CONSIDERATIONS

In summary, it is understood that surveys, evaluations and monitoring of diseases in capybaras should be carried out constantly to assess the possibility of spreading diseases or parasites to animals, or even zoonoses to people.

Studies need to provide solutions and a balance between breeding in captivity and in the natural environment in order to promote controlled or harmonious breeding between capybaras, animals and humans.

Surveys can be carried out in wild environments using camera traps, drones and/or GPS collars.

Animals killed in vehicle accidents can be a tool for assessing the health conditions of the species in a given period and area of coexistence with other species.

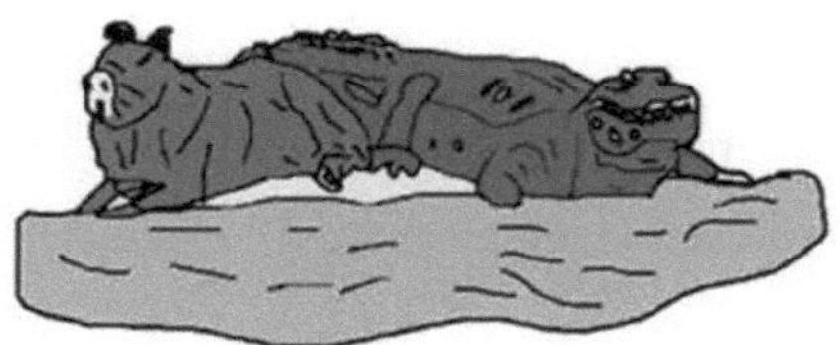

REFERENCES

ALHO, ClR. Raising and managing capybaras on small farms. - Brasília: EMBRAPA-DDT, (EMBRAPA-DPP. Documentos,13) 1986. 48p.

ALMEIDA, AR. Biondi, D. Area of use of Hydrochoerus hydrochaeris L. Cienc. anim. bras., Goiânia, v.15, n.3, p. 369-376, jul./set. 2014.

ALVES, RO. 2009. Breeding, slaughtering and commercialising wild animals. Monograph concluding the specialisation course in health surveillance and food quality control. Castelo Branco University. Brasilia, DF.

ANTONUCCI, AM and Ribeiro, TS. Commercial breeding of capybara

(Hydrochoerus hydrochaerys) in Brazil. Bibliographical review. Arch. Zootec. 63(R): 189-198. 2014. Arch. Zootec. 63(R): 189-198. 2014.

ANTUNES, JMAP. Borges, IA. Trindade, GS. Kroon, EG. Cruvinel, TMA. Peres, MG. Megid, J. Exposure of free-ranging capybaras (Hydrochoerus hydrochaeris) to the vaccinia virus. Transbound Emerg Dis. 2020;67:481-485.

CHIACCHIO, Rosely Gioia Martins Di. Health assessment of free-living capybaras (Hydrochoerus hydrochaeris) in the Cantareira region - north of São Paulo. 2012. Dissertation (Master's in Experimental and Comparative Pathology) - USP School of Veterinary Medicine and Zootechny, São Paulo, 2012.

COSTA, FB. Gerardi, M. Binder, LC. Benatti, HR. Serpa, MCA. Lopes, B. Luz, HR. Ferraz, KMPMB. Labruna, MB. Rickettsia rickettsii (Rickettsiales: Rickettsiaceae) Infecting Amblyomma sculptum (Acari: Ixodidae) Ticks and Capybaras in a Brazilian Spotted Fever- Endemic Area of Brazil. Journal of Medical Entomology, 2019, Vol. 00, No. XX. doi: 10.1093/jme/tjz141

COSTA, D.S.; Paula, T.A.R.; Fonseca, C.C. and Neves, M.T.D. 2002. Capybara reproduction. Arq Ciên Vet Zool UNIPAR, 5: 111-118.

CREED, JC. Capybara (Hydrochaeris hydrochaeris Rodentia: Hydrochaeridae): A Mammalian Seagrass Herbivore. Estuaries Vol. 27, No. 2, p. 197-200 April 2004.

DE MELO EVANGELISTA, Luanna Soares et al. Amblyomma spp. and the relationship with Brazilian spotted fever. Veterinária e Zootecnia, v. 28, p. 1-15, 2021.

DIAS TC, Stabach JA, Huang Q, Labruna MB, Leimgruber P, Ferraz KMPMB, et al. (2020). Habitat selection in natural and human-modified landscapes by capybaras (Hydrochoerus hydrochaeris), an important host for Amblyomma sculptum ticks. PLoS ONE 15(8): e0229277. https://doi.org/10.1371/journal.pone.0229277

GONZÁLEZ-Jiménez, E. 1995. The capibara. Current state of its production. FAO. Rome. Serie Estudio Producción y Sanidad Animal, 122. 112 pp.

FARIKOSKI, IO., Medeiros, LS., Carvalho, YK., Ashford, DA., Figueiredo, EES., Fernandes, DVGS., Silva, PJB., & Ribeiro, VMF. (2019). The urban and rural capybaras (Hydrochoerus hydrochaeris) as reservoir of Salmonella in the western Amazon, Brazil. Pesquisa Veterinária Brasileira, 39(1), 66-69.

FELIX, G.A. 2012. Feeding behaviour and meat quality of free-living capybara (Hydrochoerus hydrochaeris Linnaeus, 1766) in agricultural areas. Master's dissertation (Zootechnics). Federal University of Grande Dourados.

FORERO-MONTAÑA, J. Betancur, J. Cavelier, J. Hydrochaeris (Rodentia: Hydrochaeridae) in Caño Limón, Arauca, Colombia. Article in Revista de biologia tropical - July 2003.

GONÇALVES, F. Magioli, M. Bovendorp, R. S. Ferraz, K. M. P. M. B. Bulascoschi, L. et al. Moreira, MZ. Galetti, M. Prey Choice of common vampire bat (Desmodus rotundus) on an Atlantic Forest land-bridge island. Acta Chiropterologica, 22(1): 167-174, 2020.

HERREIRA, EA. Macdonald, DW. Aggression, dominance, and mating success among capybara males (Hydrochaeris hydrochaeris). Behavioural Ecology Vol. 4 No. 2.

LABRUNA M. B., Costa, F. B. Port-Carvalho, M. Oliveira, A. S. Souza, S. L. P. and Castro. M. B. Lethal Fascioliasis in Capybaras (Hydrochoerus hydrochaeris) in Brazil. American Society of Parasitologists 2018. J. Parasitol., 104(2), 2018, pp. 173-176.

LUZ HR, Costa FB, Benatti HR, Ramos VN, de A. Serpa MC, Martins TF, et al. (2019) Epidemiology of capybara-associated Brazilian spotted fever. PLoS Negl Trop Dis 13(9): e0007734.

MAGIOLIA M. Moreira, MZ. Fonseca, RCB. Ribeiro, MC. Rodrigues, MG. Ferraza, KMPMB. Human-modified landscapes alter mammal resource and habitat use and trophic structure. PNAS Latest Articles. 2019. www.pnas.org/lookup/suppl/doi:10. 1073/pnas.1904384116/-/DCSupplemental.

MENDES, A. Nogueira, SSC. Nogueira-Filho, S. A note on the cecotrophy behaviour in capybara (Hydrochaeris hydrochaeris). Article in Applied Animal Behaviour Science - February 2000.

MONES, A.; Ojasti, J. Hydrochoerus hydrochaeris Mammalian Species, No. 264, Hydrochoerus hydrochaeris. (Jun. 16, 1986), pp. 1-7.

MOREIRA JR, Ferraz KMPMB, Herrera EA, Macdonald DW. Capybara Biology, Use and Conservation of an Exceptional Neotropical Species. DOI 10.1007/978-1-4614-4000-0.

Springer. New York 2013. 424p.

NOGUEIRA, MF. Cruz, TF. Capybara diseases. Embrapa Pantanal. Corumbá, MS. 2007. 74 p. ISBN 978-85-98893-08-2.

NOGUEIRA FILHO, S.L.G. Capybara: breeding paddocks in an intensive breeding system. 2023 https://www.cpt.com.br/cursos-animais-silvestres/artigos/capivara- breeding-paddocks-in-intensive-breeding-system

PEREIRA, H. Da F. A.; Eston, M. R. De. Biology and management of capybaras (Hydrochoerus hydrochaeris) in Alberto Löfgren State Park, São Paulo, Brazil. Rev. Inst. Flor., São Paulo, v. 19, n. 1, p. 55-64, jun. 2007.

PEREIRA, FERNANDA MARA ARAGÃO MACEDO. Study of the skull of capybaras (Hydrochoerus hydrochaeris): craniometry, radiography and 3D computed tomography. 2019. 61 f.Dissertation (master's degree from UNESP). Universidade Estadual Paulista "Júlio de Mesquita Filho". Botucatu - SP.2019.

PINHEIRO, Max Silva. Capybara breeding in an intensive system. Pelotas: Embrapa Clima Temperado, (Embrapa Clima Temperado. Documentos, 200). 2007. 41 p.

RAMÍREZ-HERNÁNDEZ, A. Uchoa, F. Serpa, MCA. Binder, LC, Souza, CE. Labruna, MB. Capybaras (Hydrochoerus hydrochaeris) as amplifying hosts of

Rickettsia rickettsii to Amblyomma sculptum ticks: Evaluation during primary and subsequent exposures to R. rickettsii infection. Ticks and Tick-borne Diseases 11 (2020) 101463.

REGO, George Magno Sousa do. Investigation of trypanosomatids in free-living capybaras (Hydrochoerus hydrochaeris) in the Federal District. 2020. 72 f., il. Dissertation (Master's in Animal Sciences). University of Brasília, Brasília, 2020.

ROCHA VJ. Sekiama, ML. Gonçalves, DD. Sampieri, BR. Barbosa, GP. Dias, TC. Rossi, HR. Souza, PFP. Capybaras (Hydrochoerus hydrochaeris) and the presence of the tick (Amblyomma sculptum) on the campus of UFSCAR-Araras, São Paulo. Anim. Bras., Goiânia, v.18, 1-15, e-44671, 2017.

RODRÍGUEZ, JP. Peña, MJ. Góngora AO. Murillo RP. Obtención y evaluación del semen de capibara Hydrochoerus hydrochaeris. MVZ CÓRDOBA MAGAZINE. Volume 17(2), May - August 2012.

SANTIAGO, Claudia da Silva Leptospira spp. infection in free-living capybaras (Hydrochoerus hydrochaeris Linnaeus, 1766) in Pernambuco / Ana Claudia da Silva Santiago. - 2019. 55 f. Final Course Work (Graduation in Biological Sciences) - Federal Rural University of Pernambuco, Department of Biology, Recife, BR-PE, 2019.

SCHMIDT, SEM., and GABRIEL, EMN. Capybara: Hydrochoerus hydrochaeris (Linnaeus, 1766) - (Capybara). In: Escola do Meio Ambiente Com Vida [online]. São Paulo: Cultura Acadêmica, 2016, pp. 27-28.

STRUZA, V.S.; Machado, S.L.O.; Silva, K.S. and Santos, A.B. 2011. Forage quality of capybara grass in floodplain areas in the central region of Rio Grande do Sul, Brazil. Ciênc Rur, 41: 883- 887.

SUZUKI, C. T. The complexity of the acoustic repertoire of capybaras (Hydrochoerus hydrochaeris) 2015. 100 f. Dissertation (Master's in Psychobiology) - Ribeirão Preto School of Philosophy, Sciences and Letters, University of São Paulo, São Paulo, 2015.

VARGAS, FC. Baldi, SCV. Moro, MEG. Carrer, CRO. Population monitoring of capybaras (Hydrochaeris hydrochaeris Linnaeus, 1766) in Pirassununga, SP, Brazil. Ciência Rural, Santa Maria, v.37, n.4, p.1104-1108, jul-ago, 2007.

UIEDA, W. Septicemia by Salmonella sp in capybara (Hydrochaeris hydrochaeris). Article in Semina Ciências Agrárias - January 1995.

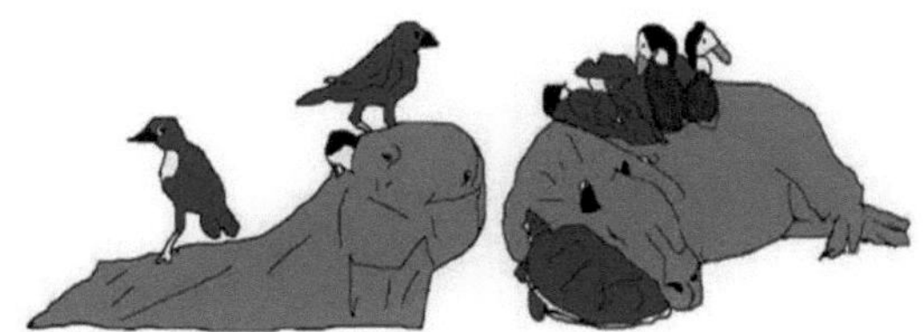

GRAPHIC ARTS CREDITS

The drawings are the work of Roberto Carlos Negreiros de Arruda, but modelled on photos or images found on the internet

CONTACT THE AUTHORS

STATE UNIVERSITY OF MARANHÃO - UEMA

Professional Postgraduate Programme in Animal Health Defence

Cidade Universitária Paulo VI, Av. Lourenço Vieira da Silva, nº 1000.

Neighbourhood: Jardim São Cristóvão, CEP 65.055-310.

Roberto Carlos Negreiros de Arruda

PhD in Animal Health Defence from UEMA and Federal Agricultural Tax Auditor from the Ministry of Agriculture and Livestock - MAPA

Federal Agricultural Superintendence of Maranhão, São Luís, MA Orcid: https://orcid.org/0000-0003-2982-6052

**Corresponding author, e-mail: rcnegreiros.arruda@gmail.com*

Daniel Praseres Chaves

Lecturer in Veterinary Medicine, State University of Maranhão, São Luís, MA

Orcid: https://orcid.org/0000-0002-5320-1469 E-mail: daniel@cernitas.com.br

Viviane Correa Silva Coimbra

Lecturer in Veterinary Medicine, State University of Maranhão, São Luís, MA

Professor at the State University of Maranhão Orcid: https://orcid.org/0000-0001-7611-6673

E-mail: vivianecorrea@yahoo.com

Francisco Borges Costa

Professor at the State University of Maranhão

Postgraduate Programme in Animal Science, State University of Maranhão, São Luís, MA

Orcid: https://orcid.org/0000-0002-6923-7183 E-mail: franc.borgesma@gmail.com

Hermes Ribeiro Luz

Professor at the Federal University of Maranhão

RENORBIO Postgraduate Programme, Federal University of Maranhão, São Luís, MA

Orcid: https://orcid.org/0000-0002-8200-6427 E-mail: hermesluz@globomail.com

Helder de Moraes Pereira

Professor at the State University of Maranhão

Postgraduate Programme in Animal Science, State University of Maranhão, São Luís, MA

Orcid: https://orcid.org/0000-0002-9354-4298 E-mail: helderpereira@professor.uema.br

José Hyrton Dantas Carneiro Júnior

State Agency for Agricultural Defence, São Luís, MA Orcid: https://orcid.org/0000-0003-4209-1169

E-mail: hyrtoncarneirojr@hotmail.com

Nádia Oliveira Medeiros

State Agency for Agricultural Defence, São Luís, MA Orcid: https://orcid.org/0000-0002-1804-4648

E-mail: nadiamedeirosvet@gmail.com

Karlos Yuri Fernandes Pedrosa

State Agency for Agricultural Defence, São Luís, MA Orcid: https://orcid.org/0000-0002-9149-6608

E-mail: mucamoyuri@hotmail.com

Valter Marchão Costa Filho

State Agency for Agricultural Defence, São Luís, MA Orcid: https://orcid.org/0000-0001-6867-0738

E-mail: vmcfilho@yahoo.com.br

Robert Ferreira Barroso de Carvalho

Municipal Health Department of Pedreira, Pedreiras/MA Orcid: https://orcid.org/0000-0002-5947-3908

E-mail: robert68vet@gmail.com

Rafael Michael Silva Nogueira

Veterinary Medicine student, State University of Maranhão, São Luís, MA Orcid: https://orcid.org/0000-0001-7694-505X E-mail: rafaelnogueira.agro@gmail.com

Mylena Andréa oliveira Torres

Professor of Medicine, Universidade Ceuma, São Luís, MA Orcid: https://orcid.org/0000-0002-5021-3130

E-mail: mylena.torres@hotmail.com

Hamilton Pereira Santos

Professor at the State University of Maranhão

Lecturer in Veterinary Medicine, State University of Maranhão, São Luís, MA

Orcid: https://orcid.org/0000-0002-6775-4056 E-mail: hpsluiza@yahoo.com.br

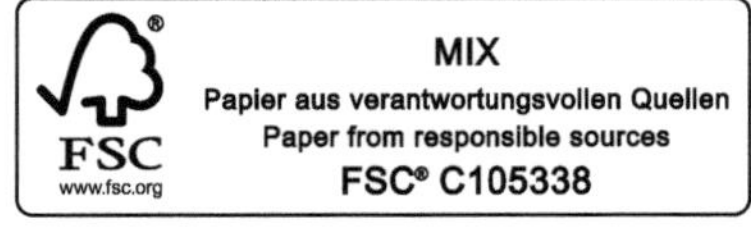

Printed by Books on Demand GmbH, Norderstedt / Germany